Make Your Skin Glow and Shine

The Best Natural Skin Care Recipes to Make Your Skin Look Beautiful Always

BY

Jenny Kings

License Notes

No part of this Book can be reproduced in any form or by any means including print, electronic, scanning or photocopying unless prior permission is granted by the author.

All ideas, suggestions and guidelines mentioned here are written for informative purposes. While the author has taken every possible step to ensure accuracy, all readers are advised to follow information at their own risk. The author cannot be held responsible for personal and/or commercial damages in case of misinterpreting and misunderstanding any part of this Book

Table of Contents

Natural Skin Care Recipes

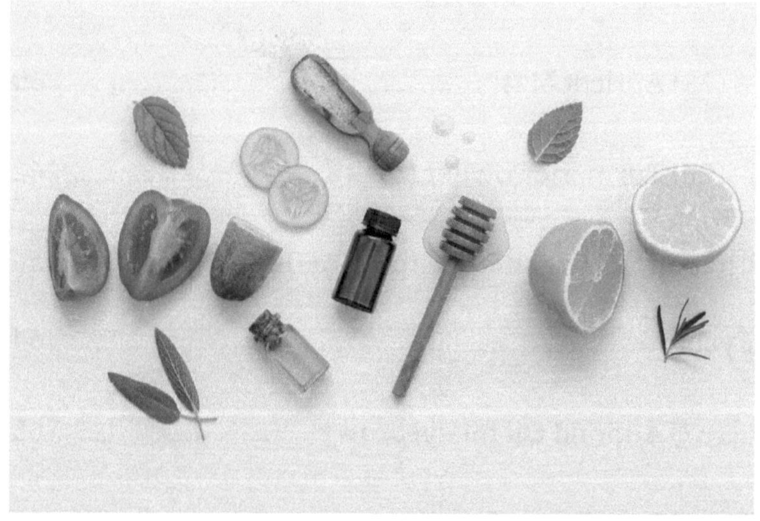

We all get panicked when we see something is wrong with our skin whether it is the face skin or the body skin. You need to know about the ways how you can keep your skin healthy to avoid any scar or mark on it. When you do not care for your skin, then it starts getting dry and causes irritation for you. The earlier you take care of it, the easier it will be for you in the future. Because as we grow old, our skin tends to be old as well. If you do not take care of it such as if you have dry skin and you do not care at all, then when you turn in old age, the cracking would start earlier than the people who took care of their skin since the beginning.

You can completely get rid of the acne if you use the natural remedies on a daily basis. You would only need to spare maximum 20 minutes of your life to get rid of acne forever. The remedies are harmless with giving you a fresh and smooth skin within one week of continuous usage. Most of the remedies contain sugar in different forms which help you in breaking the clogs and pores by removing the dead skin cells.

Know the skin type first because every human is different and their genes are different as well so not everything suits everyone. You need to know what kind of products suits you and which ingredients are best for your skin. Such as there could be some people who would not be able to keep their skin moisturized, that is because they have oily skin. Similarly, the dry skin people would not be able to survive without a lotion or cream.

Chapter I: Get Rid of Acne and Pimples with Organic Recipes

OOOOOOOOOOOOOOOOOOOOOOOOOOOOOOOOOOOOO

(1) Cinnamon Honey Mix

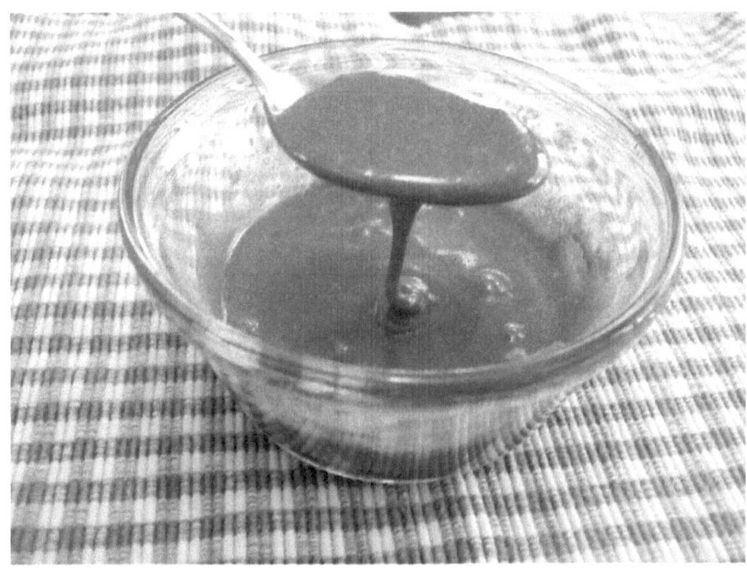

Cinnamon gives the right tone to the face by removing the dead skin cells and bringing out brighter skin tone.

List of Ingredients:

- Honey – 1 tablespoon
- Cinnamon powder – ½ teaspoons

OOOOOOOOOOOOOOOOOOOOOOOOOOOOOOOOOOOOO

Instructions:

Add a tablespoon of honey in a bowl and mix the cinnamon powder in it. Stir it well by applying it on the scar. Close your eyes and relax for a while and wash it off after 10 minutes. It will fight the clogs which are joined to release them and bring you the clear skin by vanishing the scar.

(2) Honey Mask

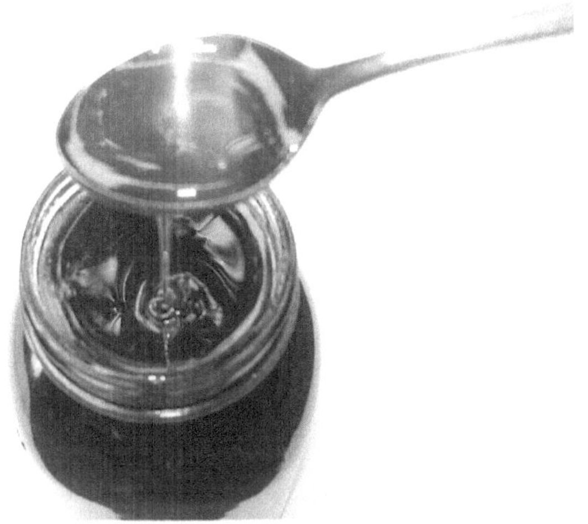

A honey mask keeps your skin fresh and healthy with its vitamin's nutrients in it.

List of Ingredients:

- Honey – 1 tablespoon
- Yogurt – 1 tablespoon

ooooooooooooooooooooooooooooooooo

Instructions:

Grab a bowl and add honey in it as well as yogurt. Mix them well together and apply it on the scar. Massage it for 10 minutes by wiping it off with a damp cloth or you can wash your face as well.

(3) Castile Face Cleanser Treatment

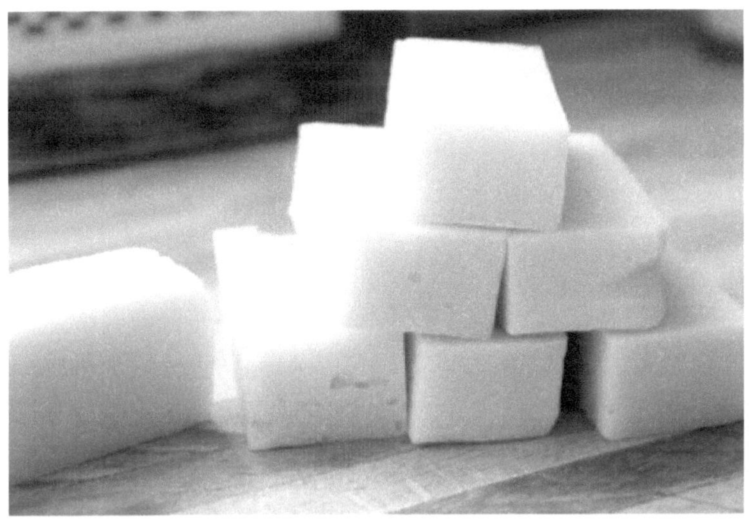

Castile is full of vitamin A and D which gives you a smooth and soft skin.

List of Ingredients:

- "Essential Oil Acne Treatment Blend" bottle (50 drops)
- Jojoba oil (¼ cup)
- Aloe Vera (¼ cup)
- Castile soap (liquid, ¼ cup)

OOOOOOOOOOOOOOOOOOOOOOOOOOOOOOOOOOOOOO

Instructions:

Take a bowl and mix jojoba oil, aloe Vera, castile soap and blend bottle together. Mix well and apply it on your face as a face cleanser. After scrubbing it for 2 minutes, wash it off.

(4) Tomato Mask for Acne Scars

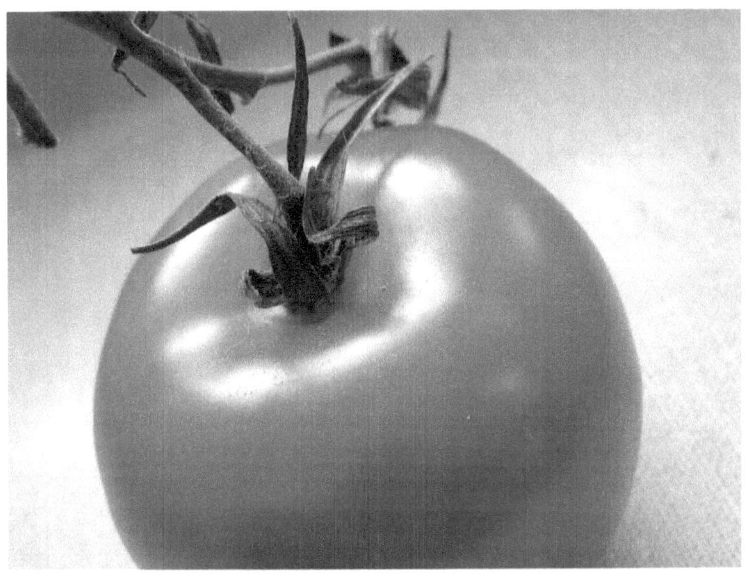

Tomato is a great source of vitamin B6 which is essential for your body to stay strong as well as keeping the skin pink.

List of Ingredients:

- Cucumber – 2
- Avocados – 2
- Tomatoes – 2

Instructions:

Cut the tomatoes, cucumbers, and avocados in half. Now take out the juice of cucumber and avocados and keep it aside. Now add the tomato's pulp in the juice. Stir it well and apply it on the face. Let it stay on the face for 20 minutes and then wash it off with water by drying it at the end.

(5) Apple Cider Mask

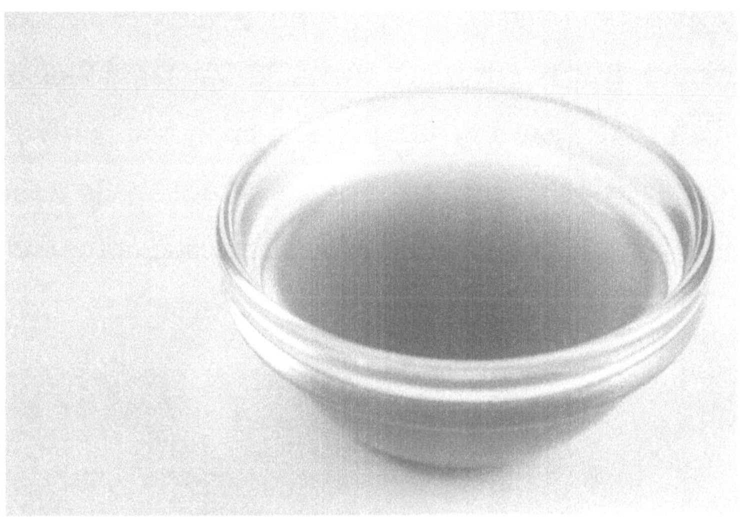

Apple cider keeps the skin glow with freshness and does not let it get dull even if you get tired by the end of the day.

List of Ingredients:

- Green tea – 2 teaspoons
- Apple cider vinegar – 1 teaspoon
- Honey – 1 teaspoon
- Sugar – 5 teaspoons

OOOOOOOOOOOOOOOOOOOOOOOOOOOOOOOOOOOOOOOO

Instructions:

Grab a bowl and a teaspoon by mixing apple cider, green tea and sugar. Stir it well until it turns into a thick texture. If it is not thick, then add few teaspoons of sugar to it. Take a cotton pad and apply the mask on your face. Massage your face to the dead cells to be removed and wash it with Lukewarm water at the end.

(6) The Face Wash Recipe

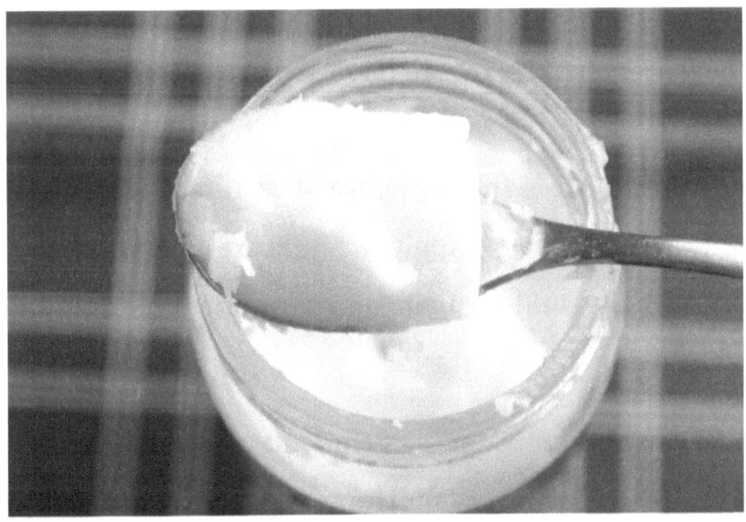

Coconut keeps your skin moisturized and does not let it produce sebum to produce pimples.

List of Ingredients:

- Coconut oil (1 tablespoon)
- Tree oil (20 drops)
- Apple Cider (1 tablespoon)
- Honey (as needed)

OOOOOOOOOOOOOOOOOOOOOOOOOOOOOOOOOOOOOOO

Instructions:

Take a bowl of plastic and add coconut oil, tree oil, apple cider and honey together. Make sure you keep the measurements correct to have good results. Mix it well with a spoon or your finger. Let it rest for about 5 minutes. During that time, wash your face with water only and dry it. Now apply the mixture with your hand on your face and scrub it for 10 minutes. Wash it and leave it damp to dry itself.

You can also make more of this mixture and store it in a bottle to use it every morning as a face wash for clear skin.

(7) Coconut Oil Remedy

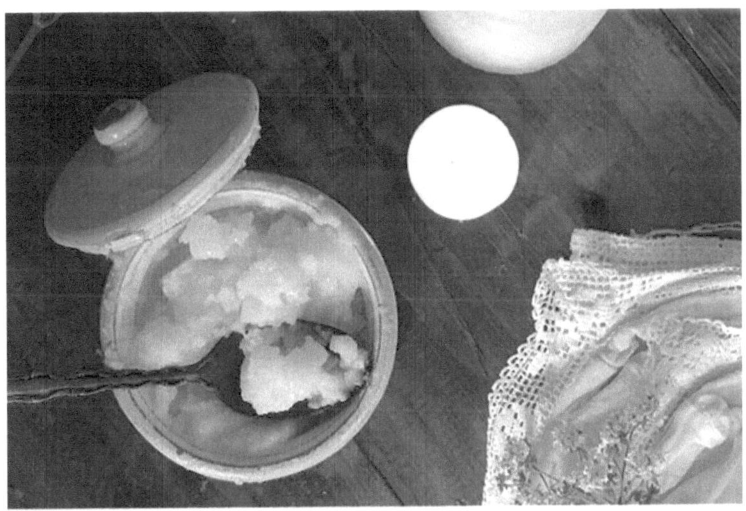

Coconut oil is a great source to keep the skin tone normal which can fight the bacteria and prevent it from producing acne.

List of Ingredients:

- Coconut oil – 1 tablespoon
- Tea tree oil – 3 drops

OOOOOOOOOOOOOOOOOOOOOOOOOOOOOOOOOOOOO

Instructions:

Mix coconut oil and tea tree oil together in a bowl and rub it on the affected area for about 2 to 3 minutes. This will ease the skin with making the scar disappear in few weeks. You need to be consistent at this. Keep the mixture in a jar and apply it every night for effective result.

(8) Herbal Face Mask for Acne Treatment

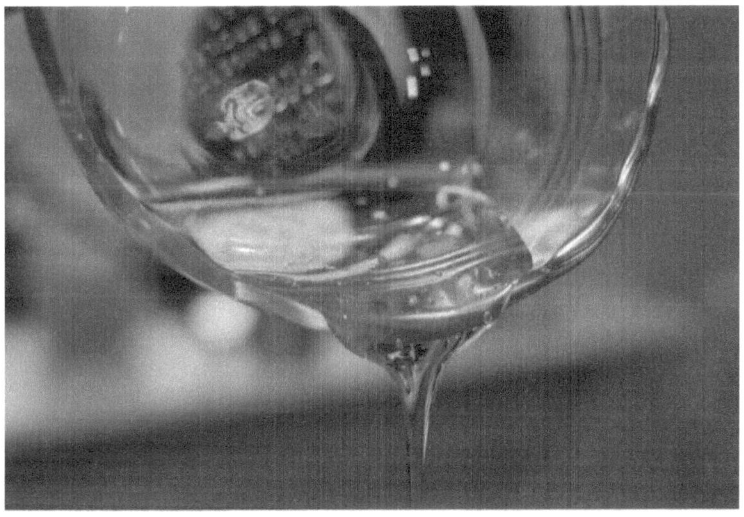

Natural ingredients made with herbals are always healing to make your skin clear and tidy.

List of Ingredients:

- "Essential Oil Acne Treatment Blend" bottle (3 drops)
- Aloe Vera (1 tsp)
- Rose petals, lavender, cinnamon, turmeric (1 teaspoon any of these powder)
- Cosmetic clay (1 teaspoon)

OOOOOOOOOOOOOOOOOOOOOOOOOOOOOOOOOOOOOO

Instructions:

Take a bowl and add blend bottle drops, Aloe Vera, cinnamon powder (or any) and cosmetic clay by making a thick paste of it. Apply the paste on your face and leave to dry for about 20 minutes. Once dried, you can wash it with Luke warm water. It will remove the acne within one week of daily application.

(9) Honey Lemon Mix for Acne Scars

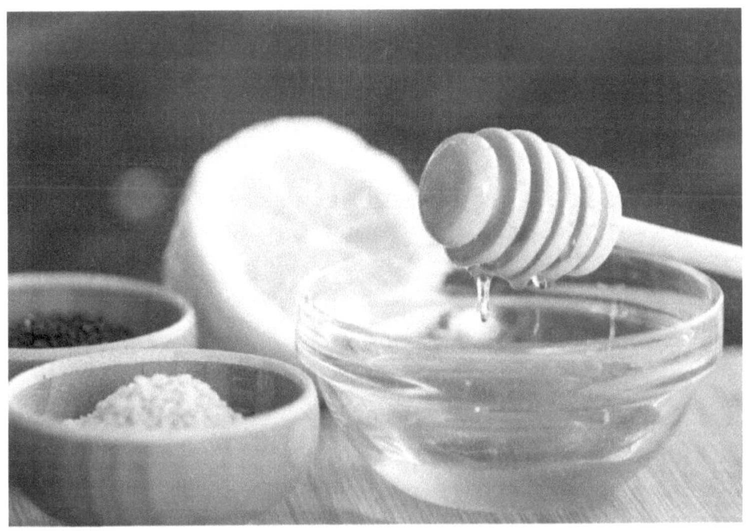

Honey and lemon make a great combination to keep the skin free of scars with providing vitamin C to the skin.

List of Ingredients:

- Lemons – 2
- Honey – 1 teaspoon

ooooooooooooooooooooooooooooooooooooooo

Instructions:

Cut the lemons in half and squeeze them completely in a bowl. Add a teaspoon of honey in and mix it well. Now grab a cotton ball and by dipping in the mixture, apply it on your face or only on the spots of acne scars. Let it stay on the face for about 10 minutes and wash it off with water by drying it at the end. Prefer doing this 2-3 times a week for improvement.

(10) Natural Acne Treatment

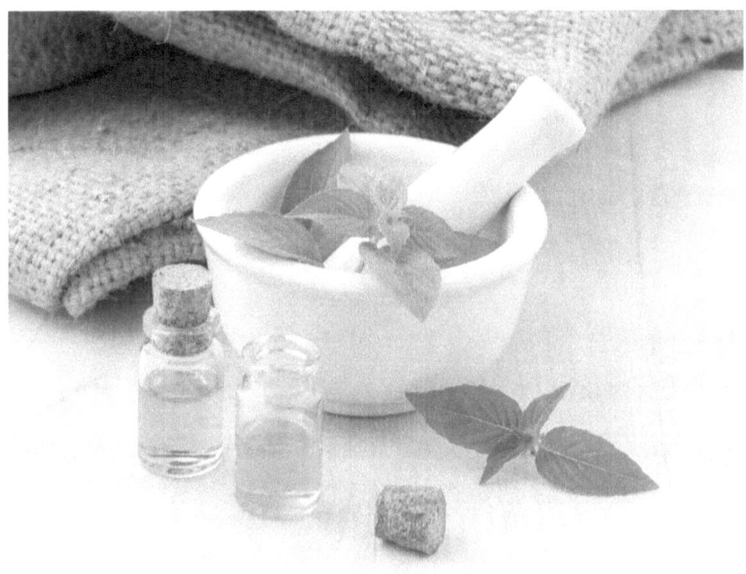

Mixture of lavender and honey keeps the skin away from dryness as well as you can get rid of pimples in no time.

List of Ingredients:

- Honey (2 tablespoons)
- Lavender oil (3 drops)
- Frankincense oil (3 drops)
- Tea tree oil (3 drops)

OOOOOOOOOOOOOOOOOOOOOOOOOOOOOOOOOOOOO

Instructions:

Arrange a bowl and add honey, lavender oil, frankincense oil and tea tree oil according to the measurements. Make a fine paste of it and apply it on your face for about 15 minutes every day. Wash it with mild cold water and dry your face with a towel.

Chapter II: Organic Recipes for Glowing Skin

OOOOOOOOOOOOOOOOOOOOOOOOOOOOOOOOOOOOOOO

(11) Oranges Whitening Skin

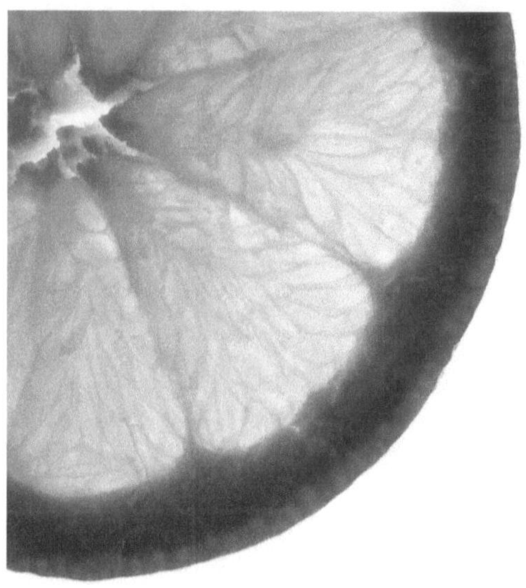

Oranges are a pure source of Vitamin C for your body. Apply it makes your skin fresh and young.

List of Ingredients:

- Orange juice (2 tablespoons)
- Turmeric (½ tablespoons)
- Cotton ball
- Water – ½ cup

Instructions:

Take a bowl and put the orange juice in it. Add the turmeric powder according to the measurements. Mix it well with the spoon and then apply it gently on the face by soaking the cotton ball in it. Keep doing it for about 20 minutes and wash it off with water. Do it daily, and you will see the difference.

(12) Honey Whitening Skin

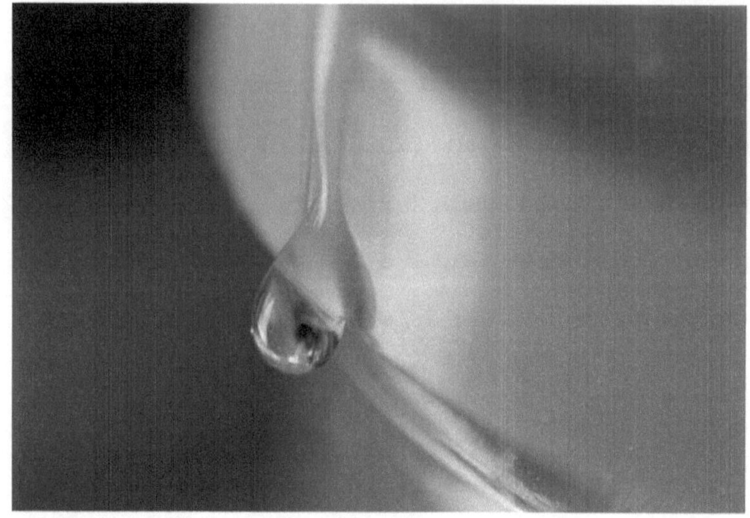

Honey whitens and smoothens the skin with leaving it smooth and soft. Removes dead skin cells and heals the skin quickly.

List of Ingredients:

- Honey (2 tablespoons)
- Lemon juice (2 tablespoons)
- Powdered milk (any, 2 tablespoons)
- Almond oil (4 drops)

OOOOOOOOOOOOOOOOOOOOOOOOOOOOOOOOOOOOOOO

Instructions:

Take a bowl and add honey, lemon juice, powdered milk and almond oil in it as per the measurements. Mix them well with a spoon and then apply it on the skin. Gently rub it and keep on doing that for 15 minutes. Honey helps the skin get brighter and smoother. Make it a habit of doing it every day to see the changes.

(13) Gram Flour

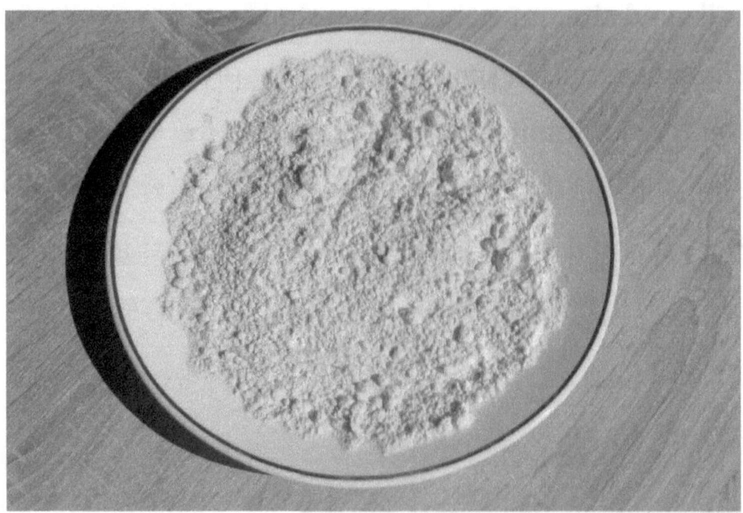

Gram flour is best to make the skin smooth, and it is rich in fiber and magnesium.

List of Ingredients:

- Gram flour (2 tablespoons)
- Rose water (3 drops)
- Almond oil (2 drops)

OOOOOOOOOOOOOOOOOOOOOOOOOOOOOOOOOOOOOOOO

Instructions:

Take a bowl and add gram flour in it as well as the rose water as required. Mix it well and now add the almond oil. Make sure it comes as a thick paste. Apply the paste on your face and wash it off once it dries. Most likely 15-20 minutes application would be enough

(14) Yogurt Whitening Skin

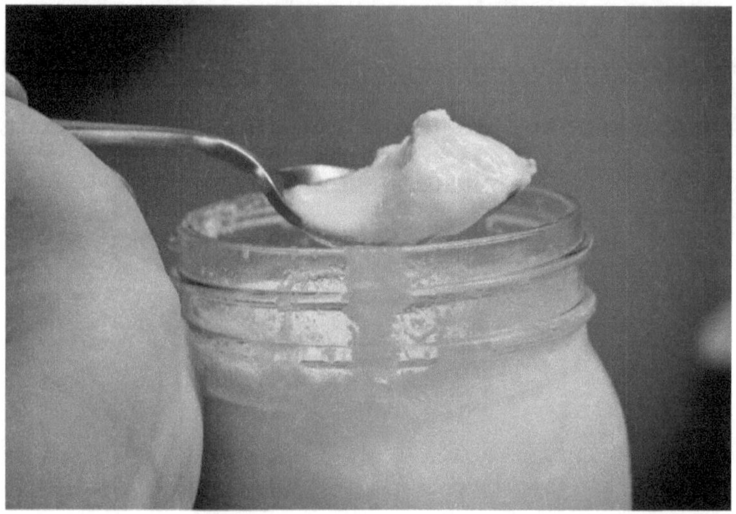

Yogurt is healthy for skin whether you eat it or apply it. It is a great source of protein.

List of Ingredients:

- Yogurt (2 tablespoons)
- Oatmeal (3 tablespoons)
- Lemon juice (1 tablespoon)
- Lavender oil as needed or (3 drops)

OOOOOOOOOOOOOOOOOOOOOOOOOOOOOOOOOOOOOOO

Instructions:

Put yogurt, oatmeal, lemon and lavender oil in a bowl and mix it well. This will turn into a paste and then apply it on your face excluding your eyes area. Gently rub it on your face skin and leave it for 15 minutes. Apply this daily for the skin tone to get equal. This will leave your skin fresh and hydrated for the day.

Chapter III: Organic Recipes for Oily, Dry and Normal Skins

oooooooooooooooooooooooooooooooooooooooo

(15) Aloe Vera Mask

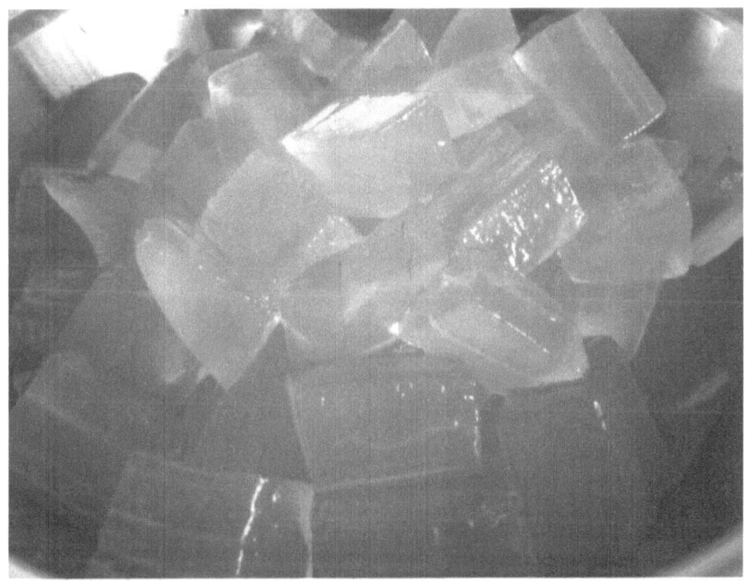

Aloe Vera gel keeps the skin moisturized even if you do not apply any lotion all the day.

List of Ingredients:

- Aloe Vera gel – 1 tablespoon
- Honey – 4 tablespoons
- Cotton balls

ooooooooooooooooooooooooooooooooooooooo

Instructions:

Mix Aloe Vera gel into honey and stir it well. Apply the mask on the face with cotton ball. Let it stay on the skin for 10 minutes and then rinse it off by patting it dry.

(16) Herbal Bath for Oily Skin

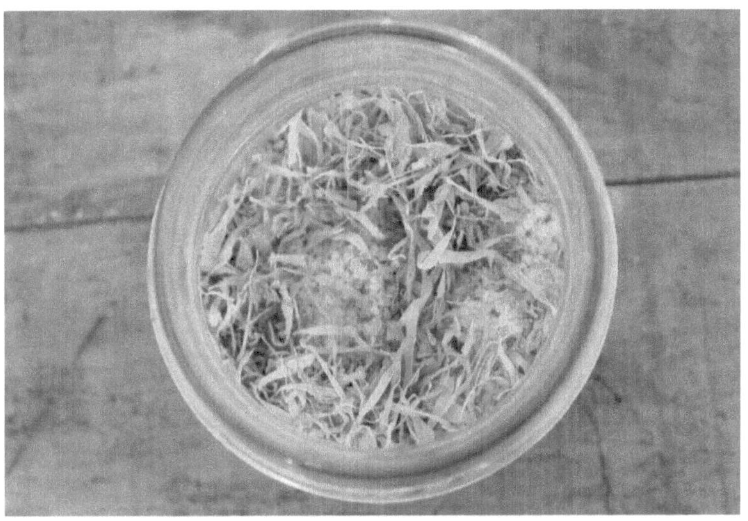

Herbal bath helps you to keep the body moisturized, so you do not need to apply lotion or any other oil after it.

List of Ingredients:

- Comfrey leaf (2 tablespoons)
- Marshmallow roots (2 tablespoons)
- Rose petals or rose water – 3 drops
- Chamomile – 2 drops

ooooooooooooooooooooooooooooooooooooo

Instructions:

Take the comfrey leaf, marshmallow roots and the chamomile in a thin cloth and mash it together. Make sure that it when you are ready to take it out; it needs to be smoothly mashed. When you take it out, put it in a bowl and add rose petals or rose water in it as needed. You can add this whole mixture in your bathtub and take a shower. It will leave a beautiful fragrance as well as your skin would be soft.

(17) Avocado Mask

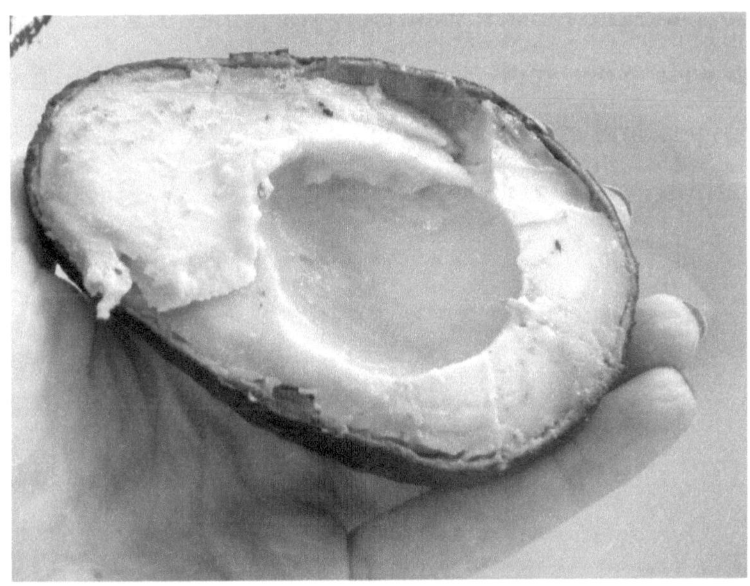

Avocado keep the skin without any spots and scars even if you have had pimples for some time. Clears all the spots on the body or face.

List of Ingredients:

- Avocado – 1 scoop
- Honey – 1 tablespoon

OOOOOOOOOOOOOOOOOOOOOOOOOOOOOOOOOOOOOOOO

Instructions:

Wash your face and pat it dry. Now, get the scoop of the avocado and mash it well. Now add honey in it and mix it well. Now apply the mask on your face with the fingers and create a thin layer of it. Wash it after 15 minutes with lukewarm water.

(18) Dandelion Leaf Remedy

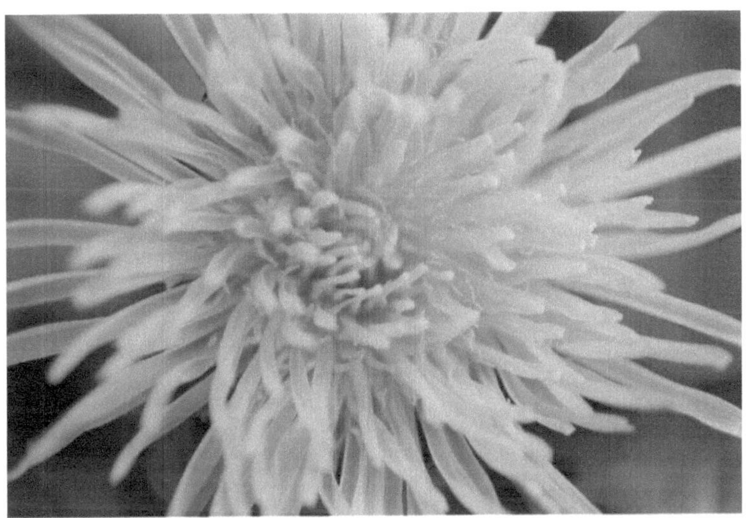

The whole body can stay fresh and smooth with the dandelion leaf remedy which can be used anytime.

List of Ingredients:

- Water – ½ cup
- Dandelion leaves (1 teaspoon)
- Almond oil (1 teaspoon)

ooooooooooooooooooooooooooooooooooooo

Instructions:

This is a quick and easy recipe for the dry skin. You need to crush the leaves first and keep them aside. On the other hand, take a pot and boil the water in it. Soak the leaves in it for about 30 minutes, then add the almond oil and mix it well. Take a bath of it. You will see how it leaves your skin moisturized.

(19) Hard Lotion for Oily Skin

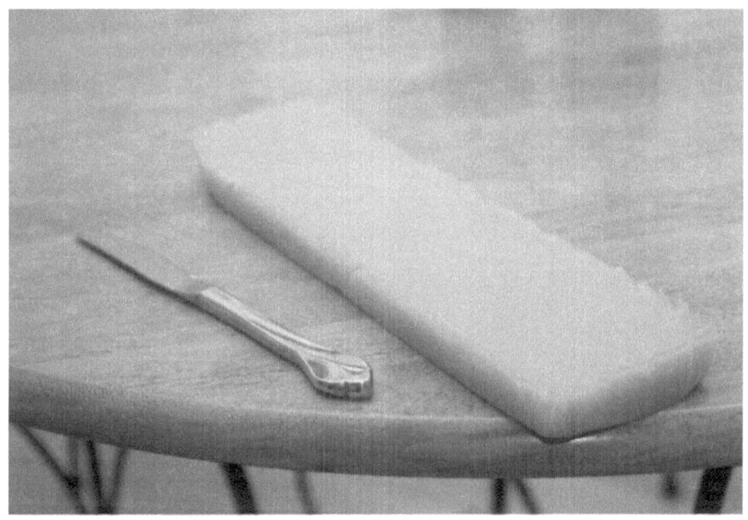

Beeswax lotion controls the oil which body produces and does not let it produce pimples.

List of Ingredients:

- Cocoa butter as needed
- Coconut oil (2 tablespoons)
- Beeswax (1 tablespoon)

OOOOOOOOOOOOOOOOOOOOOOOOOOOOOOOOOOOOOOO

Instructions:

Add cocoa butter, coconut oil and beeswax together in a bowl. It will create a mold shape. Keep it aside for about 30 minutes, and you will see it turns into hard soap. You can use it to wash your face and body which will extract the oil and leave your skin normal without even getting dried.

(20) Vanilla Cream for Dry Skin

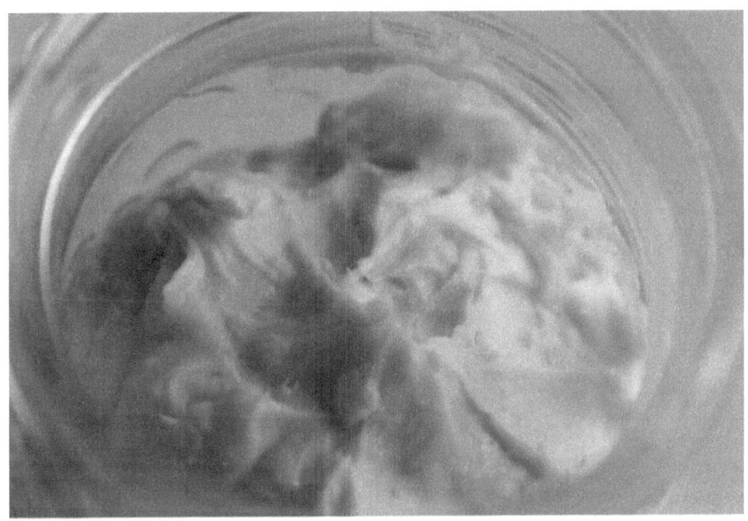

You will be able to get rid of the dryness completely with vanilla cream for dry skin recipe.

List of Ingredients:

- Shea butter (2 tablespoons)
- Coconut oil (2 tablespoons)
- Almond oil (4 tablespoons)
- Pure vanilla oil (½ tablespoons)

ooooooooooooooooooooooooooooooooooooo

Instructions:

Take a jar and add shea butter, coconut oil, almond oil and pure vanilla oil to mix it well. Keep it stored in a cool place for about 15 minutes and then apply the oil when you are done with the shower. It will leave your body soft and smooth.

Chapter IV: Organic Recipes to Protect Your Skin from Weather Effects

OOOOOOOOOOOOOOOOOOOOOOOOOOOOOOOOOOOOOOOO

(21) Banana Mask

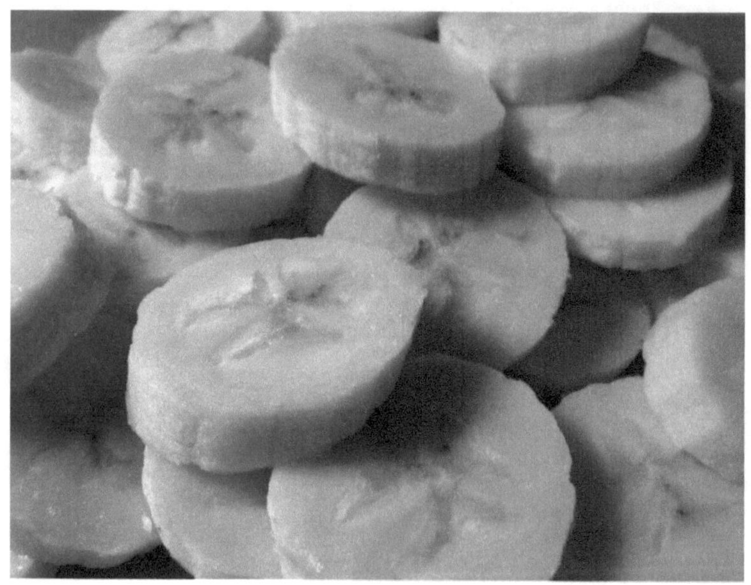

Banana mask helps you to get rid of the blackhead as well as the dryness can be managed with the moisture which it leaves on the skin.

List of Ingredients:

- Banana – 1
- Honey – 1 teaspoon
- Lemon juice – 3 drops

ooooooooooooooooooooooooooooooooooooooo

Instructions:

Peel off the banana and mash it well. Add honey in it as well as lemon juice. Mix it well and apply it on the face for 20 minutes. Rinse it off with cold water and pat it dry.

(22) Yogurt Mask

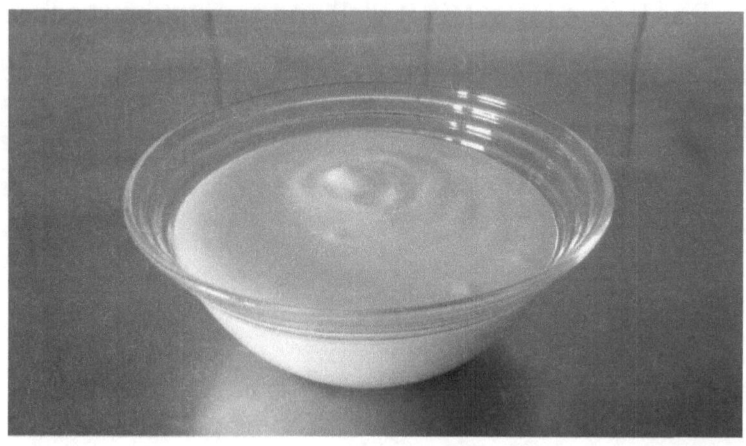

Yogurt fights the oil which can be produced in the body due to dehydration and fight during the winter season.

List of Ingredients:

- Yeast – 1 tablespoon
- Yogurt – 2 tablespoons

OOOOOOOOOOOOOOOOOOOOOOOOOOOOOOOOOOOOOO

Instructions:

Grab a bowl and add the yogurt in it by sprinkling yeast on it. Now mix it well and then apply the paste/mask on the face. Let it stay there for about 20 minutes then wash it with cold water drying it off.

(23) Cucumber Egg Mix Remedy

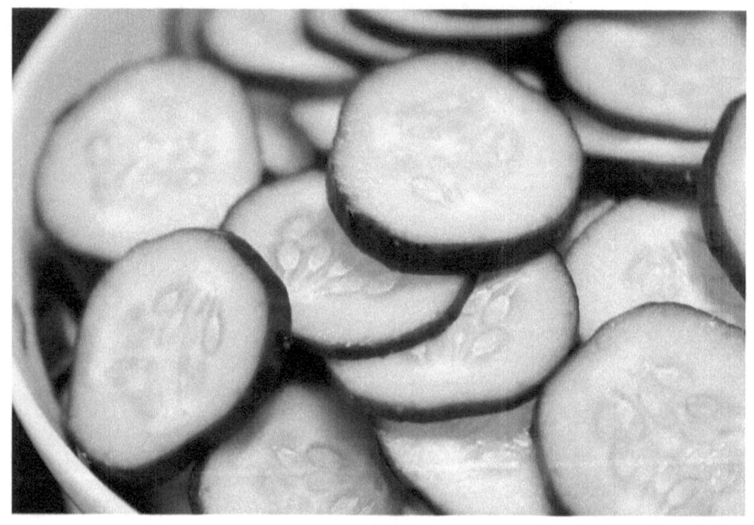

Cucumber helps skin to breathe easily with keeping it fresh and moisturized during the entire day.

List of Ingredients:

- Cucumber juice – 1 tablespoon
- Egg white – 1
- Lemon juice – 3 drops
- Clay – ½ teaspoons

ooooooooooooooooooooooooooooooooooooo

Instructions:

Mix cucumber juice, egg white, and lemon juice together in a bowl. Whisk it well and then add half teaspoon of clay making it a smooth paste. Now apply it gently on the face and let it dry for about 20 minutes. Wash it with lukewarm water and pat it dry.

(24) Egg and Lemon Mask

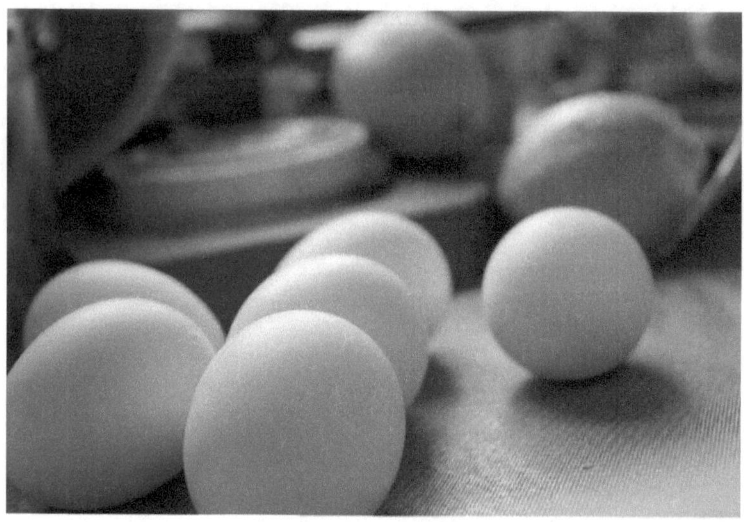

Egg is the best source of protein for your skin which keeps it fresh and clear all the time.

List of Ingredients:

- Lemon – ½ teaspoons
- Egg white – 1

OOOOOOOOOOOOOOOOOOOOOOOOOOOOOOOOOOOOOOOO

Instructions:

Break the egg in the bowl by separating the yolk from it. Now cut the lemon in half and squeeze it in the egg white. Whisk it well and then apply on the face. Leave it on the face till the morning because it will dry immediately. Simply wash the face when you wake up.

(25) Apricot Mask

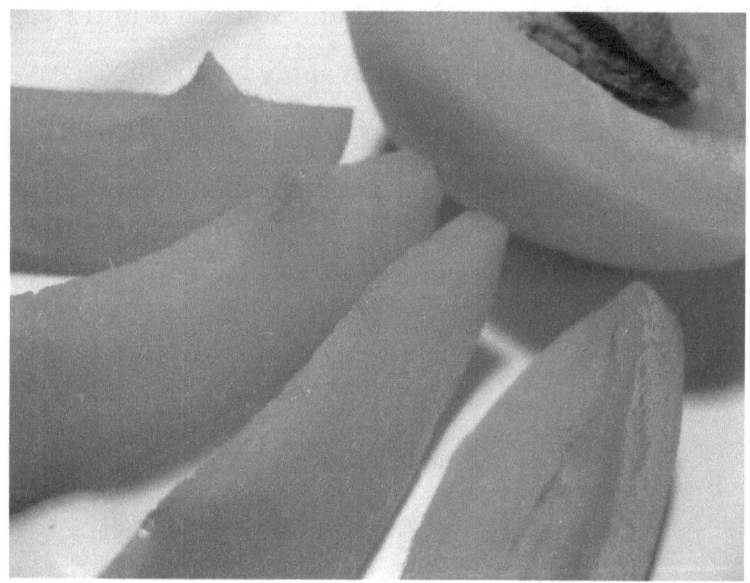

Apricot mask helps skin to stay without pimples and fresh without doing anything else but applying this mask.

List of Ingredients:

- Apricot – 1
- Yogurt – 1 tablespoon
- Clay – ½ teaspoons

ooooooooooooooooooooooooooooooooooooo

Instructions:

Peel the apricot and blend it to make a paste of it. Add yogurt to it and clay by mixing it in the blender. Pour it in a bowl and apply it on your face without covering the eyes part. Wash it off after 10 minutes for a fresh and healthy skin.

(26) Turmeric Powder Mask

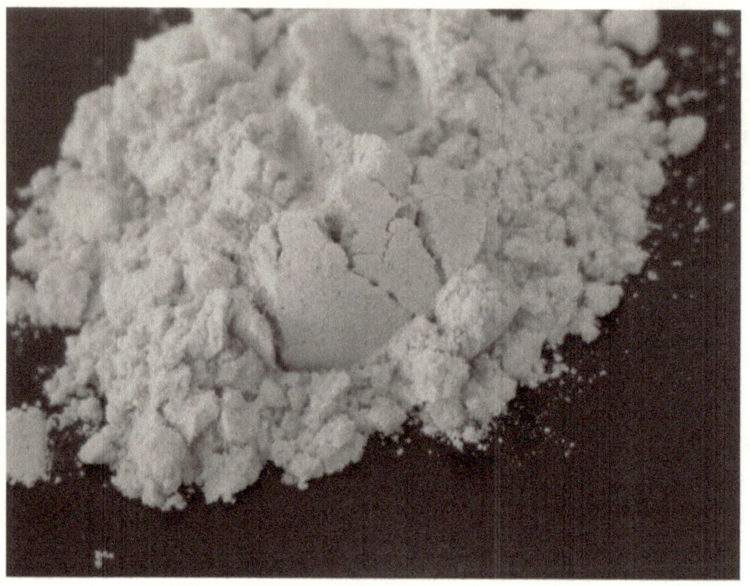

Turmeric powder keeps the skin healthy and fresh by removing the toxins and dust out from the skin.

List of Ingredients:

- Chickpea flour – ½ cup
- Turmeric powder – 2 tablespoons
- Sandalwood powder – 1 tablespoon
- Almond oil – 2 tablespoons

oooooooooooooooooooooooooooooooooooooooo

Instructions:

In a bowl, add all the ingredients such as chickpea flour, turmeric powder, sandalwood powder and almond oil by mixing it well. Make sure it makes a thick paste. Apply it on the face and keep it there for 20 minutes. Let it dry completely and wash it off with water.

Chapter V: Organic Recipes for Lips, Eyelashes, and Eyebrows

ooooooooooooooooooooooooooooooooooooooo

(27) Almond Oil for eyebrows

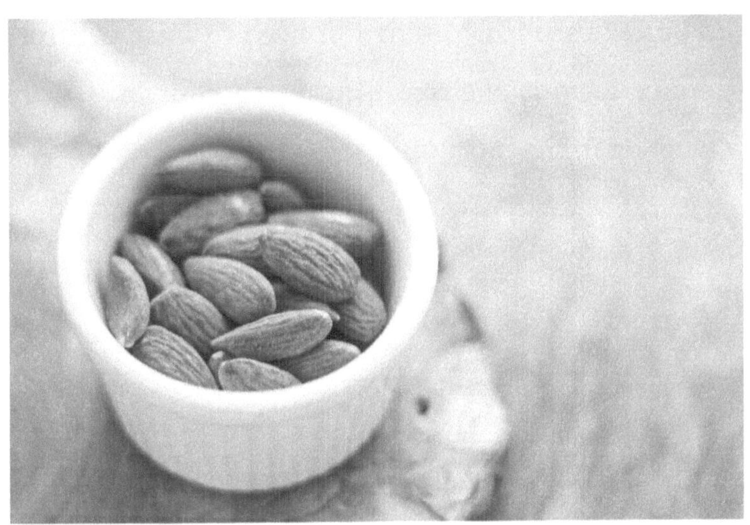

Almond oil keeps the eyebrows away from dryness with turning them into dark color with thickness as well.

List of Ingredients:

- Almond oil – 2 drops
- Rose water – 3 drops
- Vitamin E oil – 2 drops

OOOOOOOOOOOOOOOOOOOOOOOOOOOOOOOOOOOOO

Instructions:

Before sleeping, mix almond oil, rose water and vitamin E oil in the bowl and then apply it and massage it on the eyebrows. This will heal the skin from inside and outside as well. You do not need to wash it before sleeping, keep it like that. And wash your face when you get up in the morning.

(28) Rose Water for Lips

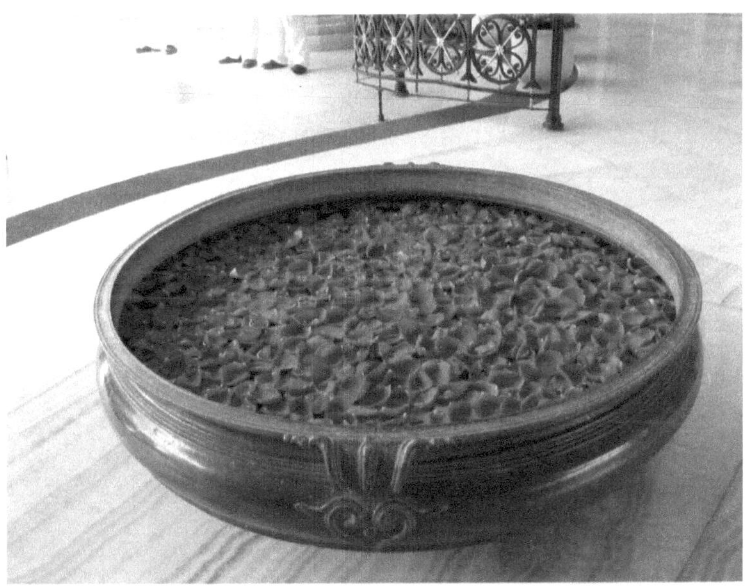

Rose water keeps the lips healthy and pinks which everyone desires by maintaining its moisture.

List of Ingredients:

- Rose water – 3 drops
- Rose petals – a bunch
- Glycerin – 3 drops
- Lavender oil – 3 drops

ooooooooooooooooooooooooooooooooooooooo

Instructions:

Add rose water, rose petals, glycerin, and lavender oil together and mix them well. Rub the mixture under your eyes for about 15 minutes. You do not need to wash it. Make sure that you do not apply makeup on top of it, so it is better that you apply that at nighttime before going to bed.

(29) Olive oil for eyelashes

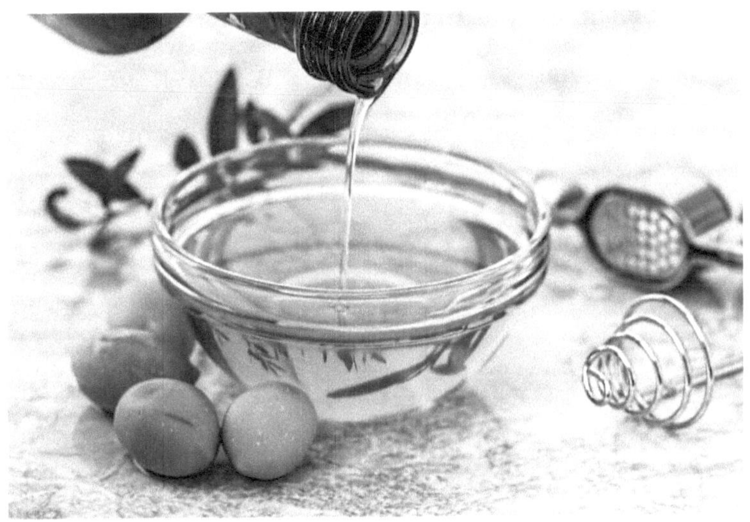

Olive oil heals the dryness or any itchiness on the eyelashes and makes them strong to grown them longer and thicker.

List of Ingredients:

- Olive oil – 2 drops
- Lavender oil – 2 drops
- Cinnamon powder – 1 teaspoon

ooooooooooooooooooooooooooooooooooooooo

Instructions:

Mix olive oil, lavender oil, and cinnamon powder together and keep it in a jar or bowl. Apply it regularly on the eyelashes either in the morning or before sleeping. Your eyelashes will turn thick and smooth without any chipping. Do it regularly to get the effective results.

(30) Rose Remedy for Lips

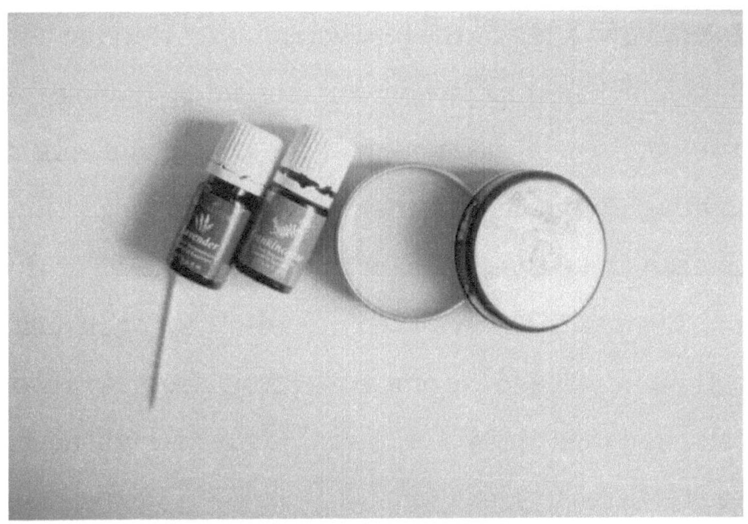

Rose and honey mix recipe do not let your lips crack even in the cold winter nights.

List of Ingredients:

- Rose water – 3 drops
- Honey (2 drops)
- Rose petal paste – 1 teaspoon
- Butter – ½ cup
- Milk cream – ½ cup
- Almond oil – 3 drops
- Saffron (one pinch)

Instructions:

Take a bowl and add the rose water in it. After that add the honey and mix it well. You should be having the rose petal paste made so melt the butter and mix it thoroughly which will make the paste thicker. Now you can add the milk cream and the almond oil at the end. Get it all together and combine it. Mix it or blend it. In the end, just add the pinch of saffron. Keep it in a cool place and then apply it on your lips anytime whenever you feel like.

Author's Afterthoughts

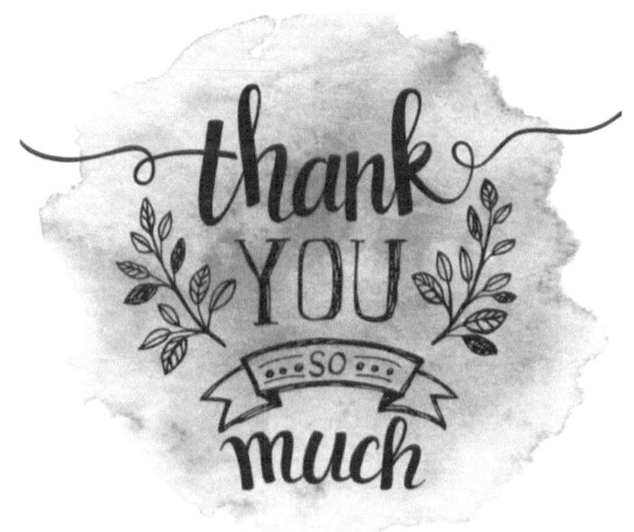

Thank you for reading my book. Your feedback is important to me. It would be greatly appreciated if you could please take a moment to REVIEW this book on Amazon so that we could make our next version better

Thanks!

Jenny Kings